GETTING YOUR MIND
TO MIND YOU!

A Beginner's Guide to Meditation for
Those Who Think They CAN'T Because
Their Mind WON'T Be Quiet!

by

Carol L Rickard, LCSW, TTS

As Featured:

DR.OZ
THE GOOD LIFE

Louisiana *radio*
network

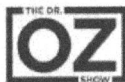

THE DR.
OZ
SHOW

esperanza
hope to cope with anxiety and depression

Doctor Health

ISBN: 978-1-947745-01-8

GETTING YOUR MIND TO MIND YOU

A Beginner's Guide to Meditation for
Those Who Think They CAN'T Because
Their Mind WON'T Be Quiet

by Carol L Rickard, LCSW, TTS

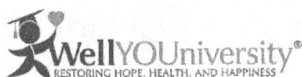

WellYOUniversity®
RESTORING HOPE, HEALTH, AND HAPPINESS

888 LIFE TOOLS (543-3866)

Carol@WellYOUniversity.com

DEDICATION

This book is dedicated to my
wonderful teacher, mentor, and friend:

Ani Trime Lhamo

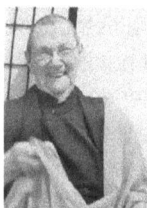

A fully ordained nun in the Tibetan Buddhist
tradition who was a longtime meditation teacher
in Princeton, N.J., and spiritual director of the
Princeton Buddhist Meditation Group.

For without you Trime, I'd have never learned
it was possible for me to meditate!

All of my love & gratitude

Contents

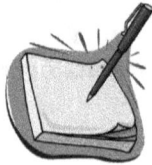

Sign up now!

To be sure to get our weekly motivational & inspirational quotes and stories!

ThePowerOfWordsEQuote.com

Why I Wrote This Book

Working in healthcare,

for years I'd always heard about how

meditation was **so good** for us…

In fact, I don't think a day went by

without hearing something being said about it

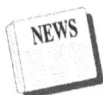 in the news or by my coworkers.

And I remember exactly what *I was thinking*

each time I'd hear it mentioned:

'Sure, it may work well for somebody else,
but NOT FOR ME!!!

***I can't get my mind* to *be quiet* -.**

There is no way, no how, that's going to happen!'

I figured pigs would be flying

before

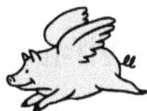

I was ever meditating!

I wished I COULD!

I saw firsthand what it could DO

&

how it could change people for the better!

I watched as it **transformed** my girlfriend.

She went from being a *highly strung & **sensitive**,*

*easily **agitated** & **stressed out** person to*

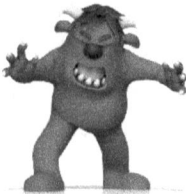

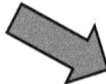

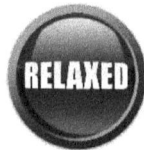

calm**, easy going, laid back, & **relaxed!

People around her noticed it too!

"What drugs are you taking?!"

they'd ask half-jokingly, half serious!

It truly was an **amazing** thing to watch!

So one day, she invited me to go with her

to her meditation group.

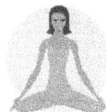

I *knew* I couldn't meditate –

but I figured I could show *my support for her*

by going with her to the center & I went!

As we got started,

her teacher - Trime said the following:

"I know some of you are new to meditation.

*I'm going to give you my **simple** instructions –*

Sit down, shut up &

see what happens!"*

I remember thinking:

'I can do that!'

And I did!

3

So can you...

This book will show you how!

Of course,

You might be *thinking to yourself **right now:***

'Okay Carol, I can sit down & shut up

BUT

*I **don't** have the TIME to meditate'*

What if I told you that it would only require

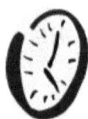

1 minute *out of your busy day?*

Could you spare **that?**

After all,

there are **1,440** of these in a day...

*Surely you could spare **one of them!***

And,

Now you might *be thinking to yourself:*

Carol, how can meditating for

1 minute a day *do any good?*

That's not long enough.

I know, it sounds ridiculous & meditation gurus will
disagree with me, but I have proof!

ME! PROOF!

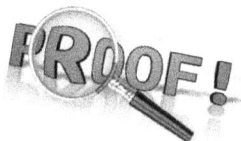

After that 1st visit to the center, I decided I would try

to **do 1 minute every day.**

My goal being to eventually **build up** to 15 minutes.

After seeing how it transformed my girlfriend,

I wanted to make a sincere attempt & see

how meditation could transform me!

I soon had my ANSWER!

You see...

My dog's had seizures since she was a puppy.

They're **grand mal** type & very **disturbing**

to watch her experience one.

Sometimes her mouth would be so wide open I

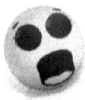

feared it would break or ***get stuck*** like that.

I'll never forget the 1st time she had a seizure

after I'd been meditating my 1 minute for 3 weeks.

I was *eerily* **calm**.....

I noticed I DIDN'T feel **disturbed**

by the seizure as I had been in the past!

I remember thinking:

"Wow, if it can create this calm in me

after just doing this little bit,

what will 15 minutes do for me?!"

Then later that same week,

I had even more evidence it was **working!**

One night at 9:00pm, my other dog, Sandy,

slipped out the front door as company was arriving -

Two things you should know:

1) I live in the *boondocks* -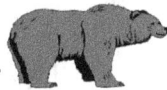

only **miles of forest** & *yes bears!*

2) And it is completely **DARK** -

there are no street lights!

7

My *normal* response:

I'D BE FREAKING OUT!!!!!

I'd get in the car and ***start driving*** up &
down the roads, trying to find her.

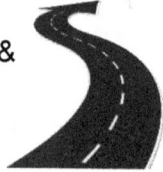

Then, I'd be **worrying** about ALL the things
that *could have happened to her….*

➢ Hit by a car (they drive reckless here)
➢ Eaten by a bear
➢ Lost in the woods & can't get back home

But there was *none* of that!

Again,

I was *strangely* **calm**!

I opened the gate to the back yard so she could

get in when she made her way home….

Not too long after that, she did!

So I know firsthand,

if you'll set aside just **1 minute** a day &

Be consistent – do it for at least 30 days in a row

You too can *notice a difference!*

The best way I like to get people to understand

how *this works* is:

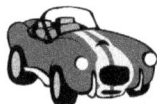

When you first start a car, and leave it in park,

the engine usually revs up & idles at a faster speed.

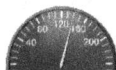

Let the car warm up & the engine rev slows down

& the car now idles at a lower speed.

I say that meditation helps

'lower the speed at which our **BRAIN** revs'

& Lowers our idle!

This leaves us…

starting off in a **calmer** place

& *less reactionary* to things that come up!

Everything I am about to share with you

I learned from my teacher:

Trime

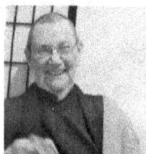

I told her I was going to write this book

to pass along the gift she'd given me.

(I wish she was still alive to see it….)

If I had NEVER heard her say:

Sit down & shut up

I don't think I would have ever tried to meditate!

You'll learn more about Trime as we go along!

There is another other way I would like you to

SEE meditation & why we all need to do it!

In his book, *Dancing with Life*, Phillip Moffitt

explained meditation the following way:

Meditation is like

doing push-ups with your *mind.*

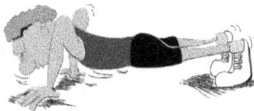

We're strengthening our

ATTENTION MUSCLES!

Which gives us the ability to

direct the focus of our thoughts

rather than

our thoughts directing us!

About This Book

I am sure by now, you have realized this ____ is

like none you have ever read before!

(Unless you have read one of my other **10** books!)

Along with **simple** & easy to understand

chapters, I tend to use a lot of pictures,

analogies, & word art

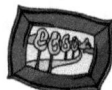

to make the information stick in the brain!

I call my approach:

SMARTheory™

It's what makes my books, programs, & services
different from all others!

KNOWLEDGE is the left brain at work.

This is where YOU *know* what to do!

Because I use "pictures" & "images", I end up
tapping in to the other side of the brain –

the right side!

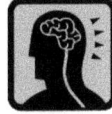

This is also the side that synthesizes things,
like the operating system in a computer!

With both sides working on the 'same page',
the end result is getting people to

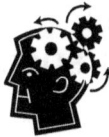

Move knowledge in to ACTION!

So, not only will you *learn*

about meditation,

you'll *USE* what you learn!

If you're not 100% satisfied when you finish reading,

let me know & I will refund your purchase price!

This book is divided in to *three parts:*

Part 1 will introduce you to some of the

Meditation Myths

Here we'll focus on dispelling the myths

that many people have about mediation

& focus on the **TRUTH!**

Holding on to these myths will actually get

in the way of **your success.**

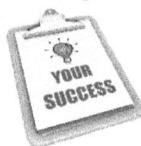

Part 2 we'll focus on **WHAT**

The goal being for you to get to KNOW

The Basics

This is what Trime was an expert at teaching!

Simple, practical, & effective

Part 3 we'll focus on **HOW** to get started.

We'll look at ways you can set yourself up for

SUCCESS!

I will introduce you to the "strategies"

I've learned & been teaching

to others for the past $2\frac{1}{2}$ years...

Lastly, I am including a

Bonus section

Here you'll find the ***secret to serenity*** &

a few gifts Trime gave me to pass along!

By the time we've made it thru all 3 parts –

You'll not only be able to **SEE** how easy it is,

You will have *already done*

your **1ST** minute!

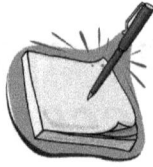

Sign up now!

To be sure to get our weekly motivational &
inspirational quotes and stories!

ThePowerOfWordsEQuote.com

Part I
Meditation Myths

Myth # 1

In order to meditate,

*you **must** make your mind quiet.*

As Trime used to say, there is only one time when

the mind will be quiet & you don't want that!

(And even then, no one's for sure!)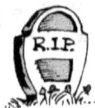

There are many different styles that exist

when it comes to meditation:

TM

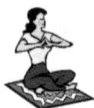 Zen

Yoga

and more....

The one I learned & am sharing with you here
DOES NOT require you mind

Be quiet!

This style is about 'seeing what your mind is doing"

WHY is this important?

Because....

WITH OUR **THOUGHTS**

WE MAKE OUR WORLD!

BUDDHA

Trime was *passionate* about getting people to

understand how our mind is

the **most** valuable asset we have!

Meditation is about being able to

TAME & **TRAIN** our mind

so we can *USE it* to our full potential.

Picture a wild horse....

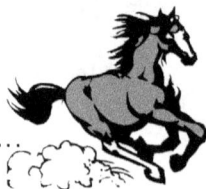

In order to be able to use this horse

there are **a couple steps** that must be taken:

Step 1) **Taming it**

Step 2) **Training it!**

Our **mind** IS *that wild horse!*

It is running around,

all over the place…

Most of the time it's running in the ▬▬

and

having a huge ▬▬ impact on our lives.

20

Meditation gives us the ability and the power to:

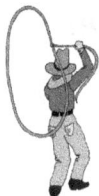

reign in our mind,

redirect it to the ✚

&

focus on our goals & successes

As you will **LEARN** in **Part 2** ,

your mind

will be anything but **quiet**

when you sit down to meditate.

Myth # 2

Meditation will leave you

feeling 'blissed out'.

Again,

think for a moment the effort that is made to

Tame & Train that horse....

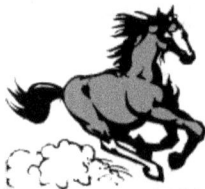

Does that leave a *blissed out* feeling?

NOT really!

It can end up feeling a little bit

more like work!

The truth is,

when we get our mind a little more

TRAINED & start to notice our thoughts –

The great majority of them are **NEGATIVE!**

Not blissful…

But as I like to say,

> YOU *DON'T KNOW*
>
> WHAT *YOU DON'T KNOW*
>
> *UNTIL YOU LEARN*
>
> **YOU DON'T KNOW IT!**
>
> CAROL L. RICKARD

Once we *KNOW* the thoughts we're thinking,

we can *then* work on changing them!!!

Myth # 3

You ***must*** meditate for

½ hour twice a day

for it to be effective

I think this will **STOP** a lot of folks from

going ahead & giving meditation a try.

I don't know about you –

But I certainly didn't have a **spare hour** to set

~~1 hour~~ aside for meditating!

Now,

I know plenty of people who've

made meditation a cornerstone of their wellness

and I certainly have great **respect** for them.

When it came to *myself* –

I determined the length of time I felt comfortable

making a commitment to was

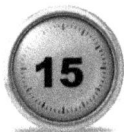

15 minutes a day!

That was my **ultimate goal!**

As we'll take a look at shortly,

that's *not how I started out!!*

In my live seminars,

At this point I like to ask:

"Raise your hand if you've *EVER* saved

"loose change"?

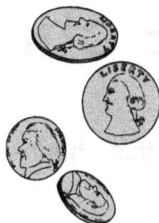

I'm talking pennies, nickels, dimes & quarters!

Usually....

Everyone's hand raises!

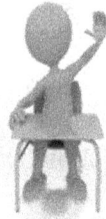

Then I ask: "What's the most money you've saved?"

So far the highest amount is $693.47!

What's the most you've saved?

So why do we go to all the trouble to save

such tiny bits of money?

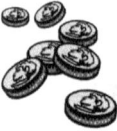 Small change

ADDs Up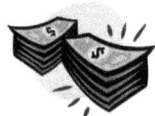

to **BIG change!**

Same thing happens here!

Small periods of time **add up** to a BIG payoff

Part II

The Basics

The Three Parts

So in the technique I learned from Trime,

there are 3 very simple parts to meditation:

Posture

Breath

Attention

A quick note about this technique:

The **formal name** is "Shamatha Vispassana"

- Shamatha means *'calm abiding'*

- Vipassana means *'insight'* or *'clear seeing'.*

This technique is used for

seeing what your mind is doing!

Imagine a glass of water with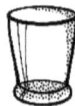

a lot of dirt stirred up inside of it.

It would be *very cloudy!*

But if you let the dirt settle – you see more clearly!

This same principle applies to our minds -

We want to *settle & see our thoughts* more clearly!

Let's start with **Posture** .

Point #1   We **MUST** be sitting *down!*

It's okay to sit in a chair -

& not on the floor!

*** We CANNOT do meditation laying down ***

When sitting in a chair –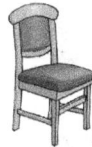

DON'T LEAN *against the back* of the chair.

Instead, we sit towards the middle to front,

with feet flat on the ground, & our back straight.

When sitting on the floor –

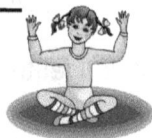

If our knees or back *start to hurt,*

It's okay to move & get ourselves comfortable!

Point #2   We **MUST** be sitting *up straight!*

We want our spine upright –

& shoulders **relaxed**.

Chin tucked in slightly.

** It's important to make sure we're not **
sitting stiff & rigid but RELAXED!

Point #3   We **CAN** rest our hands on our lap

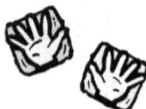   Or we can rest them on our legs!

Again, keep the shoulders relaxed.

** Some traditions hold their hands a **
special way not the case here!

Point #4   We have our eyes just slightly

EYES   open & are looking at the ground

a few feet ahead of us.

** If we find we can't do this - **
it's okay to close our eyes!

(But if we start to get sleepy —open the eyes a little!)

So here's our **Posture** one more time:

- Sitting: in chair or on floor

- Back upright

- Shoulders relaxed

- Hands on the lap

- Chin slightly tucked

- Eyes slightly open

- And jaw relaxed!!!!!

If you hurt – get **comfortable**!

If you get sleepy – *open your eyes*!

Next we have **Breath**.

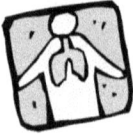

Our breath is known as

an **object** of meditation.

It is ALWAYS with us!

It is ALWAYS in *this moment*!

As Trime used to say:

"If you're not breathing in this moment, you've got a

lot more to worry about than meditation!"

Bring attention to your BREATH

Follow it as you breathe out

& it dissolves in to the air.

(like we see out breath do on a cold day!)

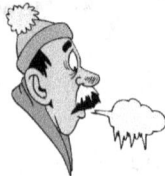

Notice it as you breathe in again.

We aren't trying to breathe IN any *special way*,

Just a normal, natural breath IN!

Again,

FOCUS attention as you breathe OUT.

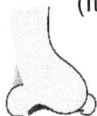

(It doesn't matter if you breathe through

your nose or your mouth....)

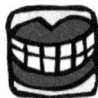

So long as you BREATHE & FOCUS on it!

As you breathe in,

notice your lungs filling with air.

LUNGS

Sometimes,

we might **need** a little help getting focused,

so one thing we can do

is to **put some words to our breath.**

33

So we can say to our self:

Breathing *in*   ***"My mind is calm"***

Breathing *out*   ***"My body is relaxed"***

Another way to **help** focus on our breath:

Count the breaths!

Breathing *in* -   **"1"**

Breathing *out* -   **"1"**

Breathing *in* -   **"2"**

Breathing *out* -   **"2"**

Breathing *in* -   **"3"**

Breathing *out* -   **"3"**

Keeping going!

I think these "word tools" are like the

training wheels I had on my bike!

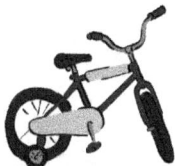

They are great getting us started

& then as our focusing ability increases,

we *may not* need to use them!

It's good to know they're there!

As you begin to get more comfortable & focused -

you can start to put a little more attention

on the **OUT BREATH.**

As it dissolves in to the atmosphere,

notice how there is a little GAP

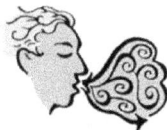

at the end just before you *naturally breath in again.*

Each time you follow the **OUT BREATH,**

continue to notice that GAP!

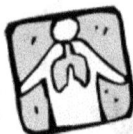

So we have 2 breathing patterns to get us started:

1) Focusing attention on both the "in" & "out" breath.

2) Focusing attention on just the "out" breath & noticing the GAP.

Next we'll look at the last of the three parts!

Attention

Soon, you'll know all that you need to start meditating!

Now we come to the 3rd part:

Attention

As we sit & focus on the breath

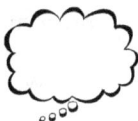

Some thoughts will pop up!

The key here is:

What we **DO** with those thoughts.

Again, we ARE NOT trying to stop them!

In fact, we need them to strengthen our

ATTENTION MUSCLES

*so our attention can go where **we put it!***

Just imagine the life you'll have

being able to **DIRECT** your attention,

instead of it directing you!

Another way I like to think of it:

Our BREATH is the anchor

that keeps us from *getting lost in our head!*

That is why, no matter where we are –

work

the store

driving

the gym

We can **always** take a moment & use our BREATH

to anchor us to a sense of calm & control!

Back to doing our meditation -

As we sit & focus on our BREATH

A thought pops up:

'I wish the dog would stop barking!'

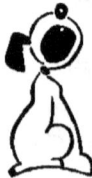

Or

'I have such a busy day ahead of me,

I don't know how I'm going to get everything done.'

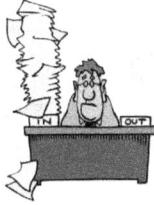

When it does - 1) Just notice it

&

2) Come back to the BREATH

We DON'T have to do anything with those thoughts!

The is to:

Just keep coming back to the BREATH!

Maybe some critical thoughts come up...

*"I'm not doing this **right**."*

*"**Why** did I think I could meditate?"*

*"This is a **waste** of time."*

Before you know it,

your mind has ***taken over*** &

you've gotten lost in thought!

Don't Worry! **It Happens!**

Which is why we don't even try to **STOP** them!

When you realize you've wandered off,

direct your attention back to the BREATH.

One of the things Trime would say:

"When you find yourself focused on thoughts
& not the BREATH, just say to yourself very gently:

'THINKING'

And focus again on the BREATH."

This is how we **TAME** & **TRAIN** our minds!

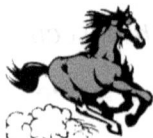

So let's review what we've covered here!

Meditation is comprised of 3 parts:

POSTURE

BREATH

ATTENTION

Our goal is to keep focused on THE BREATH

When you find yourself *thinking* & *you will* -

Gently say to yourself *'thinking'*
&
refocus on your breath.

Remember – we are strengthening our

ATTENTION MUSCLES

This is HOW we steer our lives *OFF autopilot*

& decide where it is we want to FOCUS

our attention and efforts!

I have a couple of my WordTools I'd like to share!

Here is my WordTool for FOCUS:

F_{ix}

O_{ur}

$C_{oncentration}$

U_{ntil}

$S_{uccessful!}$

Here is the one for EFFORT:

E ngage

F ull

F orce

O n

R eaching

T argets

Lastly, my WordTool for MEDITATE:

Mind

Exercise

Directing

Intention

Towards

Awareness

Thoughts

Engaged

Part III

Getting Started

So Now What?

By now, my hope is you have begun to see meditation as something you CAN DO!

And equally as important –

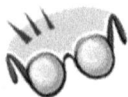

You can **SEE** why it's

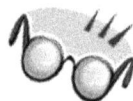

IMPORTANT to do it!

When Trime said:

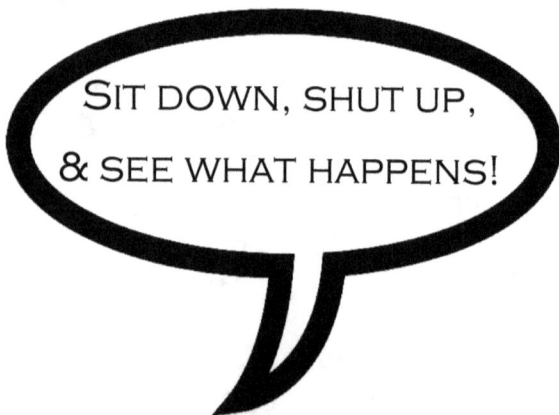

SIT DOWN, SHUT UP, & SEE WHAT HAPPENS!

She really wasn't kidding!

And that's all it takes....

I wanted to make it very easy

for you to get started....

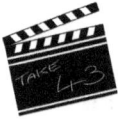

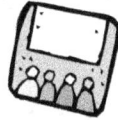

So I've made you a 1 minute meditation video
that's waiting for you at the end of this section!

This way,

the 1st time you try to meditate you

won't have to be doing it all on your own!

But before you go running off to the video,

I want to go over a few important

steps for getting started...

Step 1 - Start with making a *commitment* to do *1 minute* every day for 30 days

Step 2 - Try to do this 1 minute at the *same time* every day.

Step 3 - You must find a spot where you won't be disturbed! (bathrooms work!)

Step 4 - Set the timer on your phone to be your guide.

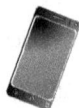

The Secret to Success:

Start off with only 1 minute!

Do this until you can focus on your BREATH

for pretty much the **whole** minute.

Even if you are using the *"training wheels"*!

Then you can *slowly* increase by 1 minute

up till you reach your desired goal.

Doing 1 minute every day

is better than

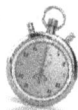

doing 10 minutes once a week!

Lastly,

Just like we can't strengthen our muscles

without doing some exercises....

We can't strengthen our

ATTENTION MUSCLES

Without doing meditation!

Reading this is only a beginning -

To watch / download the video go to

WellYOUniversity.com/Mind

What lies ahead is to

PRACTICE!

(Turn the page to see my WordTool for it!)

My WordTool is:

Purposely

Repeat

Activities

Critical

To

Improving

Core

Elements

BONUS
Section

From Stressed to Serenity

Meditation is *not* a "Magic Wand"!

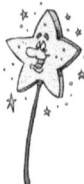

It won't immediately *move you* from

Stressed to Serenity!

However, that can come with practice!

In the meantime, I wanted to share with you a few STRESS TOOLS from my book:

"LifeTOOLS: How to Manage Life INSTEAD of Life Managing You!

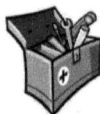

One way to eliminate A LOT of stress:

IF IT *DOESN'T* INVOLVE YOU

DON'T GET INVOLVED!

CAROL L RICKARD

Another way to think about STRESS:

IT'S NOT

WHAT HAPPENS TO YOU

HOW YOU REACT TO IT

THAT MATTERS.

EPICTETUS

I teach people to think of

STRESS as being like laundry!

It Piles Up!

There are only two ways of dealing with this "pile":

1 - AVOID adding to the pile

2 - Do a load of "*STRESS Laundry!*

"How do you do a load of **STRESS Laundry**?"

STRESS AWAY
LAUNDRY SOAP

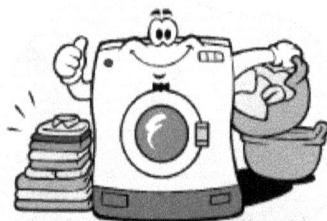

Guaranteed to lighten any day!

Directions:

* Use at least one time daily

* Separate in to piles if too
    large for one load

* May need to do multiple loads

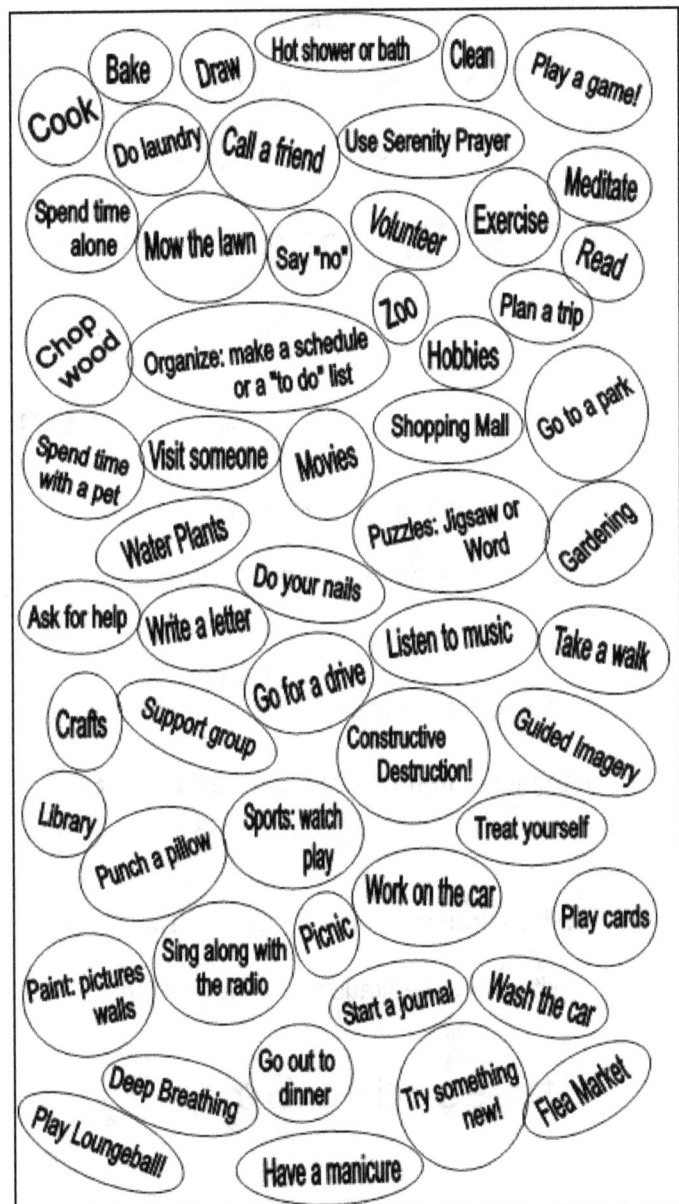

Bake

Draw

Hot shower or bath

Clean

Play a game!

Cook

Do laundry

Call a friend

Use Serenity Prayer

Spend time alone

Mow the lawn

Say "no"

Volunteer

Exercise

Meditate

Read

Chop wood

Organize: make a schedule or a "to do" list

Zoo

Hobbies

Plan a trip

Go to a park

Spend time with a pet

Visit someone

Movies

Shopping Mall

Water Plants

Puzzles: Jigsaw or Word

Gardening

Do your nails

Ask for help

Write a letter

Listen to music

Take a walk

Crafts

Support group

Go for a drive

Constructive Destruction!

Guided Imagery

Library

Punch a pillow

Sports: watch play

Treat yourself

Work on the car

Play cards

Paint: pictures walls

Sing along with the radio

Picnic

Start a journal

Wash the car

Deep Breathing

Go out to dinner

Try something new!

Flea Market

Play Loungeball!

Have a manicure

While meditation helps train us to

live in the moment, another tool

I've taught and used for **25** years is

One Day at a Time!

If you can't stay in the moment –

The next best place is **TODAY!**

Only having to deal with the STRESS

of just one day can make it *doable!*

I have an exercise I created to help people be able

to do just that: live one day at a time!

When you combine "1 Day at a Time"

with daily meditation you move from

Stressed to Serenity!

First, read the following:

YESTERDAY, TODAY, and TOMORROW

There are two days in every week that we need not worry about, two days that must be kept free from fear and apprehension.

One is **YESTERDAY**, with it's mistakes & cares, it's faults & blunders, it's aches & pains. Yesterday has passed, forever beyond our control. All the money in the world cannot bring back yesterday. We cannot undo a single   act we performed. Nor can we erase a single word we've said – Yesterday is gone!

The other day we must not worry about is **TOMORROW**, with it's impossible adversaries, it's burden, it's hopeful promise and poor performance. Tomorrow is beyond our control!

Tomorrow's sun will rise either in splendor or behind a mask of clouds – but it will rise. And until it does, we have no stake in tomorrow, for it is yet unborn.

This leaves only one day – **TODAY**. Any person can fight the battles of just one day. It is only when we add the burdens of yesterday & tomorrow that we break down.

It is not the experience of today that drives people mad—it is the remorse of bitterness for something which happened yesterday, and the dread of what tomorrow may bring.   LET US LIVE ONE DAY AT A TIME!!!!

(Author Unknown)

57

Second, take a blank piece of paper and
write Yesterday, Tomorrow, & Today on it
so it looks like this:

```
┌─────────────────────────────┐
│                             │
│          Yesterday          │
│                             │
│                             │
│                             │
│          Tomorrow           │
│                             │
│                             │
│                             │
│           Today             │
│                             │
│                             │
│                             │
└─────────────────────────────┘
```

Under "Yesterday" -

I want you to write down all the things from **the
past** (from yesterday or 20 years ago) that still
occupy your thoughts. This includes regrets,
resentments, hurts, the I shoulda-woulda-coulda's,
guilt's, & anything else that comes to mind!

<u>**Under "Tomorrow" -**</u>

I want you to write down all the things from **the future** that occupy your thoughts. Including worries, fears, "what-if's", uncertainties, hopes, & dreams!

<u>**Under TODAY -**</u>

I want you to look back over the things you've written under yesterday & tomorrow. Ask yourself this **?** about *each* of the items you have listed:

"Is there anything I can **DO** about that
TODAY?"

If there is, write down under **TODAY**
the **SPECIFIC ACTION** you can take.

It must be something you can DO!

If there isn't,
don't write anything under TODAY

Once you have completed this,
there is one last step to take!

Fold the paper *just above* where **TODAY** is written.

Now, keep folding it back & forth several times on that same crease. You can even lick it if you want but don't get a paper cut!

Now carefully tear the paper along the crease.

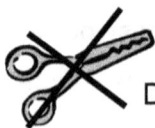

DO NOT USE SCISSORS!!!

It is IMPORTANT to do it by your own hand.

You should end up with 2 pieces of paper in your hands.

One piece has <u>Yesterday</u> & <u>Tomorrow</u> on it.

Feel free to burn this, rip it up, shred it, destroy it!

The other piece has TODAY on it.

Hold onto this!

It is the only day we *CAN* DO anything about.

You may need to do repeat this every day until you're able to focus on TODAY!

Lastly,

One of my most favorite Stress Tools:

The Serenity Prayer

GRANT ME THE SERENITY TO

ACCEPT THE THINGS
I CANNOT CHANGE

COURAGE TO CHANGE
THE THINGS I CAN

WISDOM TO
KNOW THE DIFFERENCE

My in the moment version:

Can I do anything about it

RIGHT NOW?

If so – DO IT

If NOT – Let it go!

When I told Trime I was going to write this book,
she gave me some of her affirmations to ✚ in.

These are **positive** statements we
can use once we get our meditation practice going!

Trime used to say:

"It's like planting little seeds!"

The way to use these is **simple:**

We say one sentence on our **IN BREATH**

We say the other sentence on our **OUT BREATH**

It's best to work with one affirmation at a time.

That can be 1 week or 1 month...

it's up to you!

Trime's affirmation gifts:

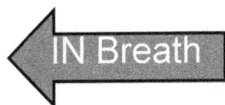

⬅ IN Breath

I cannot control what happens

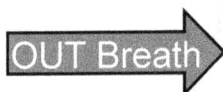

in my life

OUT Breath ➡

I can control my reactions

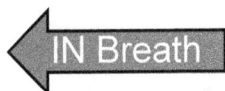

⬅ IN Breath

In this moment

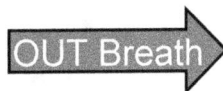

OUT Breath ➡

My life is perfect

← IN Breath

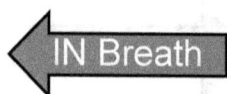

I move forward with confidence

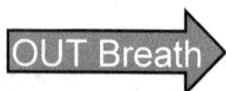

OUT Breath →

All is well in my life

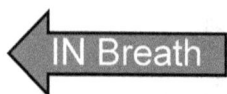

← IN Breath

I love and approve of myself

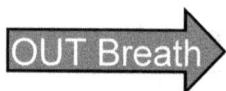

OUT Breath →

I am at peace with myself

← IN Breath

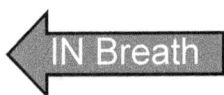

I am gentle and loving

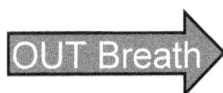

OUT Breath →

Towards myself and others

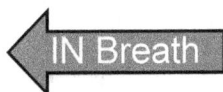

← IN Breath

I am free from pain

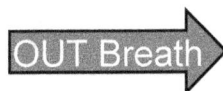

OUT Breath →

Illness and suffering

← **IN Breath**

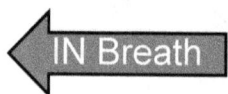

I am totally adequate

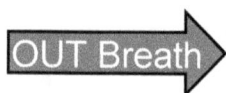

OUT Breath →

For all situations

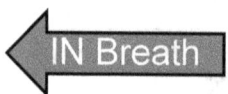

← **IN Breath**

I am stable, I am strong

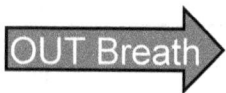

OUT Breath →

I am in control

Wrapping Things Up!

My goal in writing this book was to share with you
the gift Trime had shared with me!

Remember her **simple** instructions –

"Sit down, shut up & see what happens!"

Meditation is NOT a Magic wand

However,

When done on a consistent basis
(even 1 min.)

It can have a **magical influence** on our lives!

~ To Living Well TODAY! ~

Carol

About the Author

Carol L Rickard, LCSW, TTS, of Hopewell, NJ is founder & CEO of WellYOUniversity, LLC, a global health education company dedicated *to empowering individuals with the tools and supports to achieve lifelong wellness & recovery.*

Also known as **America's Wellness Ambassador**, Carol is a dynamic & engaging speaker who brings to life practical / useful solutions. She is a weekly contributor for Esperanza Magazine; written 13 books on stress and wellness, had a guest appearance on Dr. Oz last year

She is also the creator & host of a 30-minute wellness show on Princeton TV - **The WELL YOU Show** which can be seen at:

www.TheWELLYOUShow.com

Get more of Carol at:

Twitter: *@wellYOUlife*

"Like us" @ www.FaceBook.com/WellYOUniversity

Have Carol Speak at Your Next Event!

Get more information about how you can have Carol speak at your organization, event, or conference.

Go to: www.CarolLRickard.com

Or call: 888 Life Tools (543-3866)

Carol's Other Books

WordTools – Harnessing the Power of Words!

ANGER – A Simple & Practical Approach

Help – How to Help Those Who DON'T Want It

Selfness – Simple Self-Care Secrets

Stress Eating – How to STOP Using Food to Cope

Stretched Not Broken – Caregiver's Stress

The Caregiver's Toolbox

Transforming Illness to Wellness

Putting Your Weight Loss on Auto

The Benefits of Smoking

Moving Beyond Depression

LifeTools – How to Manage Life

Creating Compliance

Relapse Prevention

Please visit us at:

www.WellYOUniversity.com

Sign up for weekly motivational e-quote!

Check out our upcoming FREE webinars!

Learn more about our training programs.

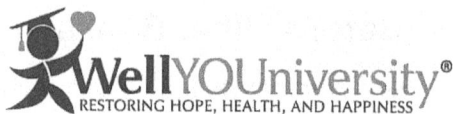

WellYOUniversity®
RESTORING HOPE, HEALTH, AND HAPPINESS

Email us your success story at:

Success@WellYOUniversity.com

We'd like to ask for your feedback

Please check out the next page
if this book has been HELPFUL for you!

We'd love to hear from you!

Feedback Card

Please take a moment & provide us some

feedback about the book you just read &

how you feel *it benefited YOU!*

_____

_____

_____

_____

Name: _____

Best Phone #: _____

Can we use your comments in our publicity materials?
Yes / No

If OK with you, what's the best time to call you:_____

Thank You!

Scan or take a picture & email:
Carol@WellYOUniversity.com

Snail mail: Carol Rickard
5 Zion Rd., Hopewell, NJ 08535

Tear along here

71